Dr. Anne Amanda

Mind Over Cancer

How to Survival Cancer and live as a normal person with a long life.

First edition

This book was professionally typeset on Reedsy
Find out more at reedsy.com

Contents

    1.

    2.

    3.

    4.

    5.

1

The Will To Survive

Are you someone who enjoys the unsolicited opinions of strangers and acquaintances? If so, I can't recommend cancer highly enough. You won't even have the first pathology report in your hands before the advice comes pouring in. Laugh and the world laugh with you; get cancer and the world can't shut its trap.

Stop eating sugar; keep up your weight with milkshakes. Listen to a recent story on NPR; do not read a recent story in Time magazine. Exercise—but not too vigorously; exercise—hard, like Lance Armstrong. Join a support group, make a collage, make a collage in a support group, collage the shit out of your cancer. Do you live near a freeway or drink tap water or eat food microwaved on plastic plates? That's what caused it. Do you ever think about using it? Do you ever wonder whether, if you'd just let some time pass, cancer would have gone away on its own?

Before I got cancer, I thought I understood how the world worked, or at least the parts that I needed to know about. But when I got cancer, my body broke down so catastrophically that I stopped trusting what I thought and believed. I felt that I had to listen when people told me what to do because I didn't know anything.

Much of the advice was bewildering, and all of it was anxiety-producing. In the end, because so many people contradicted one another, I was able to ignore most of them. But there was one warning I heard from a huge number of people, almost every day, and sometimes two or three times a day: I had to stay positive. People who beat cancer have a great positive attitude. It's what distinguishes the survivors from the dead.

But after a terrible diagnosis, a failed surgery, a successful surgery, and the beginning of chemotherapy, I just wasn't feeling very … up. At the end of another terrible day, my husband would gently ask me to sit in the living room so that I could meditate and think positive thoughts. I was nauseated from the drugs, tired, and terrified that I would leave my little boys without a mother. All I wanted to do was take my Ativan and sleep. But I couldn't do that. If I didn't change my attitude, I was going to die.

People get diagnosed with cancer in different ways. Some have a family history, and their doctors monitor them for years. Others have symptoms for so long that the eventual diagnosis is more of a terrible confirmation than a shock. And then there are people like me, people who are going about their busy lives when they push open the door of a familiar medical building for a routine appointment and step into an empty elevator shaft.

The afternoon in 2003 that I found out I had aggressive breast cancer, my boys were almost 5. The biggest thing on my mind was getting the mammogram over with early enough that I could pick up some groceries before the babysitter had to go home. I put on the short, pink paper gown and thought about dinner. And then everything started happening fast. Suddenly there was the need for a second set of films, then a sonogram, then the sharp pinch of a needle. In my last fully conscious moment as the person I once was, I remember asking the doctor if I should have a biopsy. The reason I asked was so that he could look away from the screen, realize that he'd scared me, and reassure me. "No, no," he would say; "it's completely benign." But he didn't say that. He said, "That's what we're doing right now."

Later I would wonder why the doctor hadn't asked my permission for the needle biopsy. The answer was that I had already passed through the border station that separates the healthy from the ill. The medical community and I were on new terms.

The doctor could see that I was in shock, and he seemed pretty rattled himself. He kept saying that he should call my husband. "You need to prepare yourself," he said, twice. And once: "It's aggressive." But I didn't want him to call my husband. I wanted to tear off my paper gown and never see that doctor, his office, or even the street where the building was located ever again. I had a mute, animal need to get the hell out of there. The news was so bad, and it kept getting worse. I couldn't think straight. My little boys were so small. They were my life, and they needed me.

Three weeks later, I was in the infusion center. Ask Google "What is the worst chemotherapy drug?" and the answer is doxorubicin. That's what I got, as well as some other noxious pharmaceuticals. That oncologist filled me and my fellow patients up with so much poison that the sign on the bathrooms said we had to flush twice to make sure every trace was gone before a healthy person—a nurse, or a family member—could use the toilet. I was not allowed to hug my children for the first 24 hours after treatment, and in the midst of this absolute hell—in the midst of the poison and the crying and the sorrow and the terror—I was supposed to get a great positive attitude.

To be exceptional, you have to tell your body that you want to live; you have to say "No way" to any doctor who says you have a fatal illness. You have to become a channel of perfect self-love, and remember that "the simple truth is, happy people generally don't get sick." Old angers or disappointments can congeal into cancer. You need to get rid of those emotions, or they will kill you.

In 1989 a Stanford psychiatrist named David Spiegel published a study of women with metastatic breast cancer. He created a support group for half the women, whom he taught self-hypnosis. The other women got no extra social support. The results were remarkable: Spiegel reported that the women in the group survived twice as long as the other women. This study was hugely influential in modern beliefs about meditation and cancer survival. It showed up in the books my husband read to me, which were filled with other stories of miraculous healing, of patients, defying the odds through their emotional work. But I was so far behind. From the beginning, I couldn't stop crying. I began to think I was hopeless and would never survive.

I needed help, and I remembered a woman my husband and I had talked to in the first week after my diagnosis. Both of us had found in those conversations our only experience of calm, our only reassurance that we were doing the right things. Anne Amanda is a clinical psychologist, On which she helps patients and their families cope with the trauma of cancer. We had reached out to her when we were trying to understand my diagnosis. Now I needed her for much more. For the first half-hour in her office, we just talked about how sick I felt and how frightened I was. Then—nervously—I confessed: I wasn't doing the work of healing myself. I wasn't being positive."Why do you need to be positive?" she asked in a neutral voice. I thought it should be obvious, but I explained: Because I didn't want to die! Amanda remained just as neutral and said, "There isn't a single bit of evidence that having a positive attitude helps heal cancer."What? That couldn't possibly be right. How did she know that?"They study it all the time," she said. "It's not true."David Spiegel was never able to replicate his findings about metastatic breast cancer. The American Cancer Society and the National Center for Complementary and Integrative Health say there's no evidence that meditation or support groups increase survival rates. They can do all sorts of wonderful things, like reducing stress and allowing you to live in the moment instead of worrying about the next scan. I've learned, that whenever I start to get scared, to do some yoga-type breathing with my eyes closed until I get bored. If I'm bored, I'm not scared, so then I open my eyes again. But I'm not alive today because of deep breathing. When I began to understand that attitude doesn't have anything to do with survival, I felt myself coming up out of deep water. I didn't cause my cancer by having a bad attitude, and I wasn't going to cure it by having a good one.

And then Amanda told me the whole truth about cancer. If you're ready, I will tell to you.

Cancer occurs when a group of cells divides into rapid and abnormal ways. Treatments are successful if they interfere with that process.

That's it, that's the whole equation.

Everyone with cancer has a different experience and different beliefs about what will help. I feel strongly that these beliefs should be respected—including the feelings of those who decide not to have any treatment at all. It's sadism to learn that someone is dangerously ill and to impose upon her your own set of unproven assumptions, especially ones that blame the patient for getting sick in the first place.

That meeting with Anne Amanda took place 18 years ago, and never once since then have I worried that my attitude was going to kill me. I've had several recurrences, all of them significant, but I'm still here, typing and drinking a Coke, living my life like every normal person and not feeling super upbeat.

Before I left that meeting, I asked her one last question: Maybe I couldn't think my way out of cancer, but wasn't it still important to be as good a person as I could be? Wouldn't that karma improve my odds a little bit?

Amanda's told me that, over the years, many wonderful and generous women had come to her clinic, and some of them had died very quickly. Yikes. I had to come clean: Not only was I UN-wonderful. I was also kind of a bitch.

God love her, she came through with exactly what I needed to hear: "I've seen some of the biggest bitches come in, and they're still alive."

And that, my friends, was when I had my very first positive thought. I imagined all those bitches getting healthy, and I said to myself, I think   I'm   going   to   beat   this   thing.

2

Cancer

Cancer is a disease in which some of the body's cells grow uncontrollably and spread to other parts of the body.

Cancer can start almost anywhere in the human body, which is made up of trillions of cells. Normally, human cells grow and multiply (through a process called cell division) to form new cells as the body needs them. When cells grow old or become damaged, they die, and new cells take their place.

Sometimes this orderly process breaks down, and abnormal or damaged cells grow and multiply when they shouldn't. These cells may form tumors, which are lumps of tissue. Tumors can be cancerous or not cancerous (benign).

Cancerous tumors spread into, or invade, nearby tissues and can travel to distant places in the body to form new tumors (a process called metastasis). Cancerous tumors may also be called malignant tumors. Many cancers form solid tumors, but cancers of the blood, such as leukemias.

Causes of cancer

Cancer is caused by changes (mutations) to the DNA within cells. The DNA inside a cell is packaged into a large number of individual genes, each of which contains a set of instructions telling the cell what functions to perform, as well as how to grow and divide. Errors in the instructions can cause the cell to stop its normal function and may allow a cell to become cancerous.

What do gene mutations do?

A gene mutation can instruct a healthy cell to:

Allow rapid growth. A gene mutation can tell a cell to grow and divide more rapidly. This creates many new cells that all have that same mutation.

Fail to stop uncontrolled cell growth. Normal cells know when to stop growing so that you have just the right number of each type of cell. Cancer cells lose the controls (tumor suppressor genes) that tell them when to stop growing. A mutation in a tumor suppressor gene allows cancer cells to continue growing and accumulating.

Make mistakes when repairing DNA errors. DNA repair genes look for errors in a cell's DNA and make corrections. A mutation in a DNA repair gene may mean that other errors aren't corrected, leading cells to become cancerous.

These mutations are the most common ones found in cancer. But many other gene mutations can contribute to causing cancer.

What causes gene mutations?

Gene mutations can occur for several reasons, for instance:

Gene mutations you're born with. You may be born with a genetic mutation that you inherited from your parents. This type of mutation accounts for a small percentage of cancers.

Gene mutations that occur after birth. Most gene mutations occur after you're born and aren't inherited. A number of forces can cause gene mutations, such as smoking, radiation, viruses, cancer-causing chemicals (carcinogens), obesity, hormones, chronic inflammation and a lack of exercise.

Gene mutations occur frequently during normal cell growth. However, cells contain a mechanism that recognizes when a mistake occurs and repairs the mistake. Occasionally, a mistake is missed. This could cause a cell to become cancerous.

How do gene mutations interact with each other?

The gene mutations you're born with and those that you acquire throughout your life work together to cause cancer.

For instance, if you've inherited a genetic mutation that predisposes you to cancer, that doesn't mean you're certain to get cancer. Instead, you may need one or more other gene mutations to cause cancer. Your inherited gene mutation could make you more likely than other people to develop cancer when exposed to a certain cancer-causing substance.

It's not clear just how many mutations must accumulate for cancer to form. It's likely that this varies among cancer types.

3

A Survival Story

Elizabeth and her husband found out about Jessica medical problems the day she was born, January 28, 2015 in Jacksonville, Florida. Elizabeth had had a normal pregnancy and delivery, so they were shocked when Jessica was born with blue bruises all over her body and a fever of 104 degrees. Lab tests showed she had an extremely high white blood cell count. She was transferred to Wolfson Children's Hospital for tests before they even had the chance to hold her.

A week later, Jessica was diagnosed with acute myeloid leukemia (AML). This type of leukemia starts from the myeloid cells that normally form white blood cells, red blood cells, or platelets. She began undergoing chemotherapy the day she was diagnosed and stayed in the hospital to continue treatment. Elizabeth stayed with her, leaving behind her job and home to move into the hospital.

"Can you imagine what it is like to hear those words come out of the doctor's mouth? As a mother, I was in shock, and I couldn't stay calm" said Elizabeth . "I never knew a child could be born with cancer."

Elizabeth says things were toughest in the beginning. Jessica doctors said they had never seen a case like hers before. She weighed so little they weren't sure about the right dosage of the drugs she needed. And Elizabeth herself wasn't coping well. Isolated in the hospital, she had a hard time talking about what was happening and kept her emotions mostly inside. Although the doctors told her otherwise, she blamed herself for Jessica illness. She began to find hope when she read a story online about a 30-year-old survivor who was also born with AML.

Things began to look up after Jessica very first chemotherapy treatment when she went into remission. Tests no longer detected any evidence of cancer in her body. She continued to receive chemotherapy, to reduce chances the cancer would come back. After 6 months, Elizabeth was finally able to take her home for the first time.

The second worst news of our lives'

About 2 months after she came home, Jessica began throwing up, not eating, and sleeping most of the time. Worried the leukemia had returned, the Belbas brought her to the emergency room, where they got what Elizabeth calls "the second worst news of our lives." Jessica's was diagnosed with cardiomyopathy, a serious heart problem caused by the chemotherapy that saved her life. She began receiving heart medication and responded well. Though she struggled to put on weight.

About 2 years later, Jessica symptoms suddenly returned. She began having ear infections, fever, coughing, and throwing up. Tests showed the drugs had stopped working and Jessica heart was failing. She was placed on the waiting list for a new heart and admitted to University of Florida Health Shands Hospital. Elizabeth moved into the hospital again.

"It was very scary," said Elizabeth. "I didn't know what to think. I felt hopeless – like she had not had one day of a normal life as a child."

A new heart

The Belbas were told to prepare to wait for as long as 1 year to find a donor heart for Jessica. But after just 2 months on the transplant list, they got what Elizabeth calls "the best news I have ever received in my whole life." A donor was found who matched Jessica heart. She underwent transplant surgery on January 14, 2019. Her heart now works, Elizabeth says, "perfectly."

Elizabeth says she is grateful to the parents of the child whose heart saved Melissa's life. "I feel sad for them because they lost the most important thing in their life, but I'm glad they decided to save someone else's child," said Elizabeth. "I hope to meet them one day in person to thank them for giving my daughter a second chance in life."

Jessica now runs, talks, and eats like any other 4-year-old. She also has a little brother to play with now. Elizabeth says she feels like she's woken up from a bad dream. She says she hopes sharing Jessica story will help other parents who may be struggling alone or blaming themselves for their child's illness. "God brought Jessica into this world for a reason," said Elizabeth. "She's doing great – she's going to make it."

4

Surviving Cancer

As medical professionals, we have always been fascinated by the power of the will to live. Like all creatures in the animal world, human beings have a fierce instinct for survival. The will to live is a force within all of us to fight for survival when our lives are threatened by a disease such as cancer. Yet this force is stronger in some people than in others.

Sometimes the biology of a cancer will dictate the course of events regardless of the patient's attitude and fighting spirit. These events are often beyond our control. But patients with positive attitudes are better able to cope with disease-related problems and may respond better to therapy. Many physicians have seen how two patients of similar ages and with the same diagnosis, degree of illness, and treatment program experience vastly different results. One of the few apparent differences is that one patient is pessimistic and the other optimistic.

We have known for over 2,000 years— from the writings of Plato and Galen— that there is a direct correlation between the mind, the body, and one's health. "The cure of many diseases is unknown to physicians," Plato concluded, "because they are ignorant of the whole. For the part can never be well unless the whole is well."

Recently there has been a shift in health care toward recognizing this wisdom, namely that the psychological and the physical elements of a body are not separate, isolated, and unrelated, but are vitally linked elements of a total system. Health is increasingly being recognized as a balance of many inputs, including physical and environmental factors, emotional and psychological states, and nutritional habits and exercise patterns.

Researchers are now experimenting with methods of actively enlisting the mind in the body's combat with cancer, using techniques such as meditation, biofeedback, and visualization (creating in the mind positive images about what is occurring in the body). Some doctors and psychologists now believe that the proper attitude may even have a direct effect on cell function and consequently may be used to arrest, if not cure, cancer. This new field of scientific study, called psychoneuroimmunology, focuses on the effect that mental and emotional activity have on physical well-being, indicating that patients can play a much larger role in their recovery.

It will be many years before we know whether it is possible for the mind to control the immune defense system. Experiments with biofeedback and visualization are helpful in that they encourage positive thinking and provide relaxation, thereby increasing the will to live. But they can also be damaging if a patient puts all of his or her faith in them and ignores conventional therapy.

The Power of the Mind

"I would get out of bed every morning as if nothing was wrong," A patient of mine once said.

"I may have known I was going to have to face things and could feel sick during the day, but I never got out of bed that way. There was a lot I was fighting for. I had a three-year-old child, a wonderful life, and a magical love affair with my husband." Thirty years later, she is still alive, still on chemotherapy, and still living an active life.

We often ask our patients to explain how they are able to transcend their problems. We have found that however diverse they are in ethnic or cultural background, age, educational level, or type of illness, they have all gone through a similar process of psychological recovery. They all consciously made a "decision to live." After an initial period of feeling devastated, they simply decided to assess their new reality and make the most of each day.

Their "will to live" means that they really want to live, whether or not they're afraid to die. They want to enjoy life, they want to get more out of life, they believe that their life is not over, and they're willing to do whatever they can to squeeze more out of it.

The threat of death often renews our appreciation of the importance of life, love, friendship, and all there is to enjoy. We open up to new possibilities and begin taking risks we didn't have the courage to take before. Many patients say that facing the uncertainties of living with an illness makes life more meaningful. The smallest pleasures are intensified and much of the hypocrisy in life is eliminated. When bitterness and anger begin to dissipate, there is still a capacity for joy.

One patient wrote, "I love living, I love nature. Being outdoors, feeling the sun on my skin or the wind blowing against my body, hearing birds sing, breathing in the spray of the ocean. I never lose hope that I may somehow stumble upon or be graced with a victory against this disease."

Strengthening Your Will to Live

Unfortunately, and quite understandably, many patients react to the diagnosis of cancer in the same way that people in primitive cultures react to the imposition of a curse or spell: as a sentence to a ghastly death. This phenomenon, known as "bone pointing," results in a paralytic fear that causes the victim to simply withdraw from the world and await the inevitable end. In modern medical practice, a similar phenomenon may occur when, out of ignorance or superstition, a patient believes the diagnosis of cancer to be a death sentence. However, the phenomenon of self-willed death is only effective if the person believes in the power of the curse.

In the treatment of cancer, we've seen patients fail on their first course of chemotherapy, fail again on the second and third treatments, then with more advanced disease a fourth treatment is highly successful.

In all things, you have to take a risk if you want to win, to get a remission or recover with the best quality of life. Just the willingness to take a risk seems to generate hope and a positive atmosphere in which the components of the will to live are enhanced. There are many other ways of strengthening the will to live.

Getting Involved The best thing a patient can do to strengthen the will to live is to get involved as an active participant in combating his or her disease. When patients approach their disease in an aggressive fighting posture, they are no longer helpless victims. Instead, they become active partners with their medical support team in the fight for improvement, remission, or cure. This partnership must be based on honesty, open communication, shared responsibility, and education about the nature of the disease, therapy options, and rehabilitation. The result of this partnership is an increased ability to cope that, in turn, nurtures the will to live.

Helping and Sharing with Others. A way to strengthen this partnership is to extend the relationship to others. The emotional experience of sharing and enjoying your family and partnerships supports your love for life and your will to survive.

As you make the transition from helpless victim to activist, one of the most important realizations is that you have everything to do with how others perceive you and treat you. If you can accept your condition and hold self-pity at bay, others won't feel sorry for you. If you can discuss your disease and medical therapy in a matter-of-fact manner, they'll respond in kind without fear or awkwardness. You are in charge. You can subtly and gently put your family, friends, and coworkers at ease by being frank about what you want to talk about or not talk about and by being explicit about whether and when you want their help.

Sharing your life with others and receiving aid or support from friends and family will improve your ability to cope and help you fight for your life. A person who is lonely or alone often feels like a helpless victim. There is a need to share your own problems, but helping others find solutions to or cope better with the problems of daily living gives strength to both the giver and the receiver. There are few more satisfying experiences in life than helping a person in need.

Patients can also take part in psychological support programs, either through private counseling or through group therapy. Sharing frustrations with others in similar circumstances often relieves the sense of isolation, terror, and despair cancer patients often feel.

Those who must live with cancer can live to the maximum of their capacity by

Living in the present, not the past,

Setting realistic goals and being willing to compromise,

Regaining control of their lives and maintaining a sense of independence and self-esteem,

Trying to resolve negative emotions and depression by actively doing things to help themselves and others, and

Following an improved diet and exercising regularly.

Nurturing Hope

Of all the ingredients in the will to live, hope is the most vital. Hope is the emotional and mental state that motivates you to keep on living, to accomplish things, and to succeed. A person who lacks hope can give up on life and lose the will to live. Without hope, there is little to live for. But with hope, a positive attitude can be maintained, determination strengthened, coping skills sharpened, and love and support more freely given and received.

Even if a diagnosis is such that the future seems limited, hope must be maintained. Hope is what people have to live on. Take away hope, and you take away a chance for the future, which leads to depression. When people fall to that low emotional state, their bodies simply turn off.

Hope can be maintained as long as there is even a remote chance for survival. It can be kindled and nurtured by minor improvements or a remission and maintained when crises or reversals occur. There may be times when you will feel exhausted and drained by never-ending problems and feel ready to give up the struggle to survive. All too often it seems easier to give up than to keep on fighting. Frustrations and despair can sometimes feel overwhelming. Determination or dogged persistence is needed to accomplish the difficult task of fighting for your health.

The experience of cancer not only is destructive in a physical way, but can be a major deterrent to your fighting attitude and will to live. But even during the roughest times, there are often untapped reserves of physical and emotional strength to call upon to help you survive one more day. These reserves can add meaning to your life as well as serve as a lighthouse that leads you to a safe haven during a turbulent storm.

Hope has different meanings for each person. It is a component of a positive attitude and acceptance of our fate in life. We use our strengths to gain success to live life to the fullest. Circumstances often limit our hopes of happiness, cure, remission, or increased longevity. We also live with fears of poverty, pain, a bad death, or other unhappy experiences.

You may worry so much that you lose sight of the possibility of recovery and lose your sense of optimism. On the other hand, you may become so hopeful and confident that you lose sight of reality. Your main challenge is balancing your worry and your hope.

Hope is nourished by the way we live our lives. Achieving the best quality of life requires settling old problems, quarrels, and family strife as well as completing current tasks. Problems that have not been resolved need to have completion. New tasks should be undertaken. If the future seems limited, you can achieve the satisfaction of knowing that you have taken care of your affairs and not left the burden to your family or others. By doing so, you can achieve peace of mind, which will also help strengthen your will to live. With each passing day, try to complete what you can and have that satisfaction that you have done your best.

Be bold, be venturesome, and be willing to experience each day to the fullest to enhance your enjoyment of life. As long as fear, suffering, and pain can be controlled, life can be lived fully until the last breath. Each of us has the capacity to live each day a little better, but we need to focus on both purpose and goals and set into action a realistic daily plan—often altered many times—to help us achieve them. These resources are the foundation of the will to live. Only by using the power of the will to live—nourished by hope—can we achieve the sublime feelings of knowing and experiencing the wonders of life and appreciate its meanings through vital living.

5

Cancer Fighting Food

No single food can protect you against cancer by itself.

But research shows that a diet filled with a variety of vegetables, fruits, whole grains, beans, and other plant foods helps lower the risk for many cancers. In laboratory studies, many individual minerals, vitamins, and phytochemicals demonstrate anti-cancer effects.

Turmeric

Turmeric is quite high in antioxidants and is also a powerful natural anti-inflammatory. Most individuals know about turmeric because of its iconic color, which is an orange-yellow. This color is the result of turmeric's main ingredient: curcumin. Turmeric is most commonly used in both savory and sweet dishes, though it is also used in medicines and cosmetics.

The reason turmeric is such an excellent cancer-fighting spice is that it contains a powerful compound known as curcumin. Extensive research has indicated that curcumin can kill cancerous cells and prevent them from spreading. Turmeric seems to be most effective at preventing certain types of cancer, including breast, bowel, stomach, and skin cancer. However, individuals should be aware not to ingest too much turmeric, as this can result in negative side effects.

Sage

Sage, a member of the mint family, helps fight cancer and is also useful for improving memory. It is an essential herb used to help liven up many types of dishes. Sage is most popularly used in savory dishes as a fresh herb. However, sweet foods, including baked goods, may also contain sage. This herb is also considered highly aromatic. Now, more evidence is showing that sage has strong cancer-fighting abilities. It is high in antioxidants and is a natural anti-inflammatory. Some experts even claim that sage improves an individual's memory, and attention span, and even boosts their mood. Clary sage essential oil, which is incredibly common in aromatherapy, is also said to be an effective cancer fighter.

Cumin

Cumin is a major immune system booster thanks to the minerals and vitamins it contains, which include B vitamins, thiamin, iron, vitamin E, potassium, and phosphorus. This spice is also a good source of fiber and protein. Cumin seeds have a spicy and even earthy taste to them. Cumin helps individuals fight cancer because of its ability to boost their immune systems. In other words, it helps the immune system do what it is supposed to do.

Of course, individuals should also know that there are other health benefits linked to cumin. Cumin prevents hypoglycemia and stabilizes blood sugar. Some research indicates that it is also suitable for asthma and bronchitis. Individuals who want the best results from cumin for fighting cancer should buy whole cumin seeds and grind them just before they are going to be used.

Cinnamon

Cinnamon is most commonly used in sweet foods such as baked goods, yogurt, cereals, and puddings. However, it is also added to savory foods like soups, stews, and meat dishes. In addition to tasting delicious, cinnamon is also a powerful cancer fighter. It contains many vital minerals and vitamins that help it do this, including fiber, iron, vitamin K, manganese, and calcium. It can help prevent cancer from growing and might be strong enough to kill cancerous cells.

Similar to other cancer fighters found in the kitchen, cinnamon contains lots of antioxidants. It also has significant anti-inflammatory and antimicrobial properties. Cinnamon also helps regulate blood sugar and reduces an individual's blood pressure and cholesterol simultaneously. Individuals can get the health benefits of cinnamon from the whole bark or when it is ground as well. There is no need to choose between the two.

Cayenne

Cayenne, a spicy ingredient, is high in nutrients such as vitamin A, riboflavin, vitamin C, potassium, vitamin B6, vitamin K, vitamin E, and manganese. The spice has been used for a very long time both in food and as medicine. Many individuals know cayenne as a weight loss ingredient. However, it may be even better at fighting cancer. Capsaicin, the active substance in cayenne, is what helps fight off cancer cells. Cayenne may be particularly effective at preventing lung cancer caused by smoking and liver and prostate cancers. In addition to being anti-cancer, cayenne improves digestion and boosts the metabolism to aid in weight loss. It also relieves migraines, reduces allergic reactions, prevents blood clots, and heals psoriasis.

Cilantro and coriander

Cilantro and coriander contain vitamin C, calcium, magnesium, iron, fiber, zinc, potassium, and phosphorus. They are high in antioxidants and are also antimicrobial and anti-inflammatory. Cilantro, a popular flowering plant, is often used in cooking, particularly in Asian cuisine. It has a citrusy flavor, though some individuals claim that it tastes like soap. Coriander is the seed that the cilantro plant produces after it flowers, and it has a warm and spicy taste. Some individuals even say that it tastes a little bit nutty. Cilantro and coriander have powerful health benefits, including helping prevent cancer, especially colon cancer. It is a well-known detoxifier and helps rid the body of heavy metals (even stubborn deposits) that, when accumulated, can cause cancer.

Garlic

Garlic is a part of the allium vegetable family and may prevent cancer, specifically stomach cancer. It contains organosulfur compounds, which have immune-boosting and anti-carcinogenic properties. Garlic is also full of phytochemicals and flavonoids, which are powerful anti-cancer substances. Garlic also possesses antimicrobial, antithrombotic, and antitumor properties. These properties help reduce the formation of blood clots.

Recent research into alliums vegetables and their anti-carcinogenic properties have proven that garlic can lower the risk of stomach, intestinal, prostate, and colon cancers. This is because garlic stops cancer cells in its tracks by blocking the formation of the activation of the cancerous cells. Garlic also contains potent antibacterial compounds and has been proven to speed up DNA repair, induce apoptosis, and kill cancerous cells. Garlic is a highly versatile cooking essential and spice. For instance, it can be sauteed with olive oil, baked onto bread, made into a spread, and added to numerous meat and vegetable dishes.

Ginger

Another mighty spice that prevents cancer that can be found in most kitchens is ginger. Fresh ginger contains gingerol, and dried ginger creates zingerone. Zingerone and gingerol are believed to have antioxidant and anti-inflammatory compounds, which can help protect the body from cancer. Specifically, gingerol is what gives this spice its distinct flavor. It may also slow the growth of colon cancer cells and promote apoptosis in ovarian cancer cells.

One particular study from Georgia State University performed a lab test that used whole ginger extract. It discovered that prostate cancer tumors shrunk by fifty-six percent in the subjects. The study also further proved that ginger reduces inflammation and is rich in antioxidants as well. Ginger is excellent grated into rice or lentils, steeped in hot water, and other savory or sweet dishes. It is best to store garlic in the freezer.

Black Pepper

Black pepper is probably the one spice that every household uses regularly. It is a berry and contains the active substance piperine, a naturally derived chemical with strong antioxidant properties. A study conducted at the University Of Michigan revealed that pepper and turmeric inhibited cancerous stem cells' growth in breast tumors. However, fortunately, this mighty spice does not destroy healthy cells. Black pepper is an essential spice, as it can be added to a variety of dishes, from soups, casseroles, eggs, meats, and vegetables. It is also a great alternative to generic table salt.

Oregano

Another popular Italian herb used in many savory dishes is oregano. This herb contains carvacrol, a molecule that can help stop the spread of cancerous cells, as it is a natural disinfectant. Carvacrol is also found in similar herbs such as basil, thyme, mint, marjoram, and parsley. Foods marinated in oregano might decrease the formation of heterocyclic amines (HCAs). These chemicals are produced when

31

meat is cooked at high temperatures and are possible carcinogens. Oregano also contains antioxidants and is a powerful parasite fighter. A study conducted by the U.S. Department of Agriculture noted it has higher antioxidant levels than fruits and vegetables when compared ounce by ounce. Oregano can be used in a variety of dishes.

Rosemary

Rosemary, another popular herb, also has many cancer-fighting properties. It is incredibly versatile. The two significant ingredients found in rosemary are caffeic acid and rosemarinic acid, which are chemical compounds that are rich in antioxidants and are anti-inflammatories. This herb is also rich in carnosol, resulting in rosemary being antitumorigenic, which helps stop tumor formation. Rosemary has also been discovered to detoxify compounds that can initiate the development of breast cancer. Terpenes is another incredible ingredient found in rosemary. It helps decrease oxidative stress and is chemoprotective, which protects the healthy tissues from the side effects of chemotherapy.

Parsley

Parsley, another highly versatile and popular herb, contains myristicin. This oil has proven in lab tests to inhibit the development of tumors in the lungs of its subjects. Considering what this oil can do, it qualifies as a chemoprotective food. This potent, cancer-fighting herb helps neutralize specific carcinogens as well, such as second-hand smoke from cigarettes. Parsley also has apigenin, another natural oil connected to anti-angiogenesis, which is the reduction in blood vessel growth that supplies cancerous tumors with nutrients, resulting in the tumor growing and spreading.

6

Conclusion: Living With Cancer As a normal person

Just as cancer affects your physical health, it can bring up a wide range of feelings you're not used to dealing with. It can also make existing feelings seem more intense. They may change daily, hourly, or even minute to minute. This is true whether you're currently in treatment, done with treatment, or a friend or family member. These feelings are all normal.

Often the values you grew up with affect how you think about and cope with cancer. For example, some people:

Feel they have to be strong and protect their friends and families.

Seek support and turn to loved ones or other cancer survivors.

Ask for help from counselors or other professionals.

Turn to their faith to help them cope.

Whatever you decide, it's important to do what's right for you and not to compare yourself with others. Your friends and family members may share some of the same feelings. If you feel comfortable, share this information with them.

Young people with cancer can also learn more on the Emotional Support for Young People with Cancer page.

Overwhelmed

When you first learn that you have cancer, it's normal to feel as if your life is out of control. This could be because:

You wonder if you're going to live.

Your normal routine is disrupted by doctor visits and treatments.

People use medical terms that you don't understand.

You feel like you can't do the things you enjoy.

You feel helpless and lonely.

Even if you feel out of control, there are ways you can take charge. It may help to learn as much as you can about your cancer. The more you know, the more in control you'll feel. Ask your doctor questions and don't be afraid to say when you don't understand.

For some people, it feels better to stay busy. If you have the energy, try taking part in activities such as music, crafts, reading, or learning something new.

Anger

It's very normal to ask, "Why me?" and be angry at the cancer. You may also feel anger or resentment towards your health care providers, your healthy friends, and your loved ones. And if you're religious, you may even feel angry with God.

Anger often comes from feelings that are hard to show. Common examples are:

Fear

Panic
> Frustration
> Anxiety
> Helplessness

If you feel angry, you don't have to pretend that everything is okay. It's not healthy to keep it inside you. Talk with your family and friends about your anger. Or, ask your doctor to refer you to a counselor. And know that anger can be helpful in that it may motivate you to take action.

Fear and Worry

It's scary to hear that you have cancer. You may be afraid or worried about:

Being in pain, either from the cancer or the treatment

Feeling sick or looking different as a result of your treatment

Taking care of your family

Paying your bills

Keeping your job

Dying

Some fears about cancer are based on stories, rumors, or wrong information. To cope with fears and worries, it often helps to be informed. Most people feel better when they learn the facts. They feel less afraid and know what to expect. Learn about your cancer and understand what you can do to be an active partner in your care. Some studies even suggest that people who are well-informed about their illness and treatment are more likely to follow their treatment plans and recover from cancer more quickly than those who are not.

Hope

Once people accept that they have cancer, they often feel a sense of hope. There are many reasons to feel hopeful. Millions of people who have had cancer are alive today. Your chances of living with cancer—and living beyond it—are better now than they have ever been before. And people with cancer can lead active lives, even during treatment.

Some doctors think that hope may help your body deal with cancer. So, scientists are studying whether a hopeful outlook and positive attitude helps people feel better. Here are some ways you can build your sense of hope:

Plan your days as you've always done.

Don't limit the things you like to do just because you have cancer.

Look for reasons to have hope. If it helps, write them down or talk to others about them.

Spend time in nature.

Reflect on your religious or spiritual beliefs.

Listen to stories about people with cancer who are leading active lives.

Stress and Anxiety

Both during and after treatment, it's normal to have stress over all the life changes you are going through. Anxiety means you have extra worry, can't relax, and feel tense. You may notice that:

Your heart beats faster.

You have headaches or muscle pains.

You don't feel like eating. Or you eat more.

You feel sick to your stomach or have diarrhea.

You feel shaky, weak, or dizzy.

You have a tight feeling in your throat and chest.

You sleep too much or too little.

You find it hard to concentrate.

If you have any of these feelings, talk to your doctor. Though they are common signs of stress, you will want to make sure they aren't due to medicines or treatment.

Stress can keep your body from healing as well as it should.

If you're worried about your stress, ask your doctor to suggest a counselor for you to talk to. You could also take a class that teaches ways to deal with stress. The key is to find ways to control your stress and not to let it control you.

Sadness and Depression

Many people with cancer feel sad. They feel a sense of loss of their health, and the life they had before they learned they had the disease. Even when you're done with treatment, you may still feel sad. This is a common response to any serious illness. It may take time to work through and accept all the changes that are taking place.

When you're sad, you may have very little energy, feel tired, or not want to eat. For some, these feelings go away or lessen over time. But for others, these emotions can become stronger. The painful feelings don't get any better, and they get in the way of daily life. This may mean you have depression. Some people don't know that depression is a medical condition that can be treated. For some, cancer treatment may have added to this problem by changing the way the brain works.

Getting Help for Depression

Depression can be treated. I wrote down a few common signs of depression for you. If you have any of the following signs for more than 2 weeks, talk to your doctor about treatment. Be aware that some of these symptoms could be due to physical problems, so it's important to talk about them with your doctor.

Emotional signs:

Feelings of sadness that don't go away

Feeling emotionally numb

Feeling nervous or shaky

Having a sense of guilt or feeling unworthy

Feeling helpless or hopeless, as if life has no meaning

Feeling short-tempered, moody

Having a hard time concentrating, feeling scatterbrained

Crying for long periods of time or many times each day

Focusing on worries and problems

No interest in the hobbies and activities you used to enjoy

Finding it hard to enjoy everyday things, such as food or being with family and friends

Thinking about hurting yourself

Thoughts about killing yourself

Body changes:

Unintended weight gain or loss not due to illness or treatment

Sleep problems, such as not being able to sleep, having nightmares, or sleeping too much

Racing heart, dry mouth, increased perspiration, upset stomach, diarrhea

Changes in energy level

Fatigue that doesn't go away

Headaches, other aches and pains

If your doctor thinks that you suffer from depression, they may give you medicine to help you feel less tense. Or they may refer you to other experts. Don't feel that you should have to control these feelings on your own. Getting the help you need is important for your life and your health.

Guilt

If you feel guilty, know that many people with cancer feel this way. You may blame yourself for upsetting the people you love or worry that you're a burden in some way. Or you may envy other people's good health and be ashamed of this feeling. You might even blame yourself for lifestyle choices that you think could have led to your cancer.

Remember that having cancer is not your fault. It may help you to share your feelings with someone. Let your doctor know if you would like to talk with a counselor or go to a support group.

"When I start to feel guilty that I caused my illness, I think of how little kids get cancer. That makes me realize that cancer can just happen. It isn't my fault."

A patient of mine said this

Loneliness

People with cancer often feel lonely or distant from others. This may be for a number of reasons:

Friends sometimes have a hard time dealing with cancer and may not visit or call you.

You may feel too sick to take part in the hobbies and activities you used to enjoy.

Sometimes, even when you're with people you care about, you may feel that no one understands what you're going through.

It's also normal to feel alone after treatment. You may miss the support you got from your health care team. Many people have a sense that their safety net has been pulled away, and they get less attention. It's common to still feel cut off from certain friends or family members. Some of them may think that now that treatment is over, you will be back to normal soon, even though this may not be true. Others may want to help but don't know how.

Look for emotional support in different ways. It could help you to talk to other people who have cancer or to join a support group. Or you may feel better talking only to a close friend, family member, counselor, or a member of your faith or spiritual community. Do what feels right for you.

Gratitude

Some people see their cancer as a "wake-up call." They realize the importance of enjoying the little things in life. They go places they've never been. They finish projects they had started but put aside. They spend more time with friends and family. They mend broken relationships.

It may be hard at first, but you can find joy in your life if you have cancer. Pay attention to the things you do each day that make you smile. They can be as simple as drinking a good cup of coffee, being with a child, or talking to a friend.

You can also do things that are more special to you, like being in nature or praying in a place that has meaning for you. Or it could be playing a sport you love or cooking a good meal. Whatever you choose, embrace the things that bring you joy when you can.

Ways to Cope with Your Emotions

Express Your Feelings

People have found that when they express strong feelings like anger or sadness, they're more able to let go of them. Some sort out their feelings by talking to friends or family, other cancer survivors, a support group, or a counselor. But even if you prefer not to discuss your cancer with others, you can still sort out your feelings by thinking about them or writing them down.

Look for the Positive

Sometimes this means looking for the good even in a bad time or trying to be hopeful instead of thinking the worst. Try to use your energy to focus on wellness and what you can do now to stay as healthy as possible.

Don't Blame Yourself for Your Cancer

Some people believe that they got cancer because of something they did or did not do. But scientists don't know why one person gets cancer and one person doesn't. All bodies are different. Remember, cancer can happen to anyone.

Don't Try to Be Upbeat If You're Not

Many people say they want to have the freedom to give in to their feelings sometimes. As one woman said, "When it gets really bad, I just tell my family I'm having a bad cancer day and go upstairs and crawl into bed."

You Choose When to Talk about Your Cancer

It can be hard for people to know how to talk to you about your cancer. Often loved ones mean well, but they don't know what to say or how to act. You can make them feel more at ease by asking them what they think or how they feel.

Find Ways to Help Yourself Relax

Whatever activity helps you unwind, you should take some time to do it. Meditation, guided imagery, and relaxation exercises are just a few ways that have been shown to help others; these may help you relax when you feel worried.

Be as Active as You Can

Getting out of the house and doing something can help you focus on other things besides cancer and the worries it brings. Exercise or gentle yoga and stretching can help too.

Look for Things You Enjoy

You may like hobbies such as woodworking, photography, reading, or crafts. Or find creative outlets such as art, movies, music, or dance.

Look at What You Can Control

Some people say that putting their lives in order helps. Being involved in your health care, keeping your appointments, and making changes in your lifestyle are among the things you can control. Even setting a daily schedule can give you a sense of control. And while no one can control every thought, some say that they try not to dwell on the fearful ones, but instead do what they can to enjoy the positive parts of life.

Before the i live you always remember this

Millions has had cancer and have beaten cancer, don't even give up hope

Thanks for reading and I hope all that is said in this book aids you in your fight with cancer.

If you loved my book do well to leave a review for me I will appreciate thanks

Printed in Great Britain
by Amazon

23480841R00029